T0144927

The Sweet Miracle of XYLITOL

The Sweet Miracle of XYLITOL

FRAN GARE, N.D.

Basic Health
PUBLICATIONS, INC.

The information contained in this book is based upon the research and personal and professional experiences of the author. It is not intended as a substitute for consulting with your physician or other health-care provider. Any attempt to diagnose and treat an illness should be done under the direction of a health-care professional.

The publisher does not advocate the use of any particular health-care protocol but believes the information in this book should be available to the public. The publisher and author are not responsible for any adverse effects or consequences resulting from the use of the suggestions, preparations, or procedures discussed in this book. Should the reader have any questions concerning the appropriateness of any procedures or preparation mentioned, the author and the publisher strongly suggest consulting a professional health-care advisor.

Basic Health Publications, Inc.

ISBN: 978-1-59120-038-3 (Pbk.)
ISBN: 978-1-68162-819-6 (Hardcover)

Editor: Christopher Mariadason
Typesetter/Book design: Gary A. Rosenberg
Cover design: Mike Stromberg

Contents

Foreword

With industrialization of the planet, refined sugar in the form of sucrose (cane or table sugar) and fructose (corn and fruit sugar) has made its way into the human diet in relatively large amounts. These sugars had traditionally been consumed as unrefined constituents of whole natural foods. Today, due to the industrialization of growing and refining food, we are inundated with sugar-rich commercial food products that are quite different from the foods our ancestors ate.

The human race has demonstrated a limited ability to slowly evolve genetically to cope with changes in environment and food supply over many millennia. For example, the Eskimos, a robust people, have historically thrived primarily on animal-based foods. Brahmans from India, who are of a different genetic stock, have thrived on a vegetarian diet. Neither group does well on the fast and packaged food of the Standard American Diet (SAD). This diet is actually fraught with health hazards for everyone regardless of heritage.

Food is being genetically engineered and chemically altered for profit by commercial interests with disregard for the long-term health of the consumer. Such adulteration of food accelerates development of chronic diseases such as dental cavities, obesity, diabetes, cancer, hardening of the arteries, and hypertension. Humans cannot genetically adapt fast enough to the commonplace, artificial changes in our diets imposed by commercial interests.

When I was a child, I watched a fair amount of television. Tony the Tiger was my mentor. I was too young to know better. I ate cornflakes so saturated with sugar toppings that it had a frosting. Sugar in such a form and quantity reduces the immune competence of white blood cells. As a child, I had my share of sinus and tonsil infections. I had rampant cavities. My dentist had lots of business drilling my teeth and filling them with toxic metals. Cereal not supersaturated with sugar would not do. I looked forward to eating sugar-frosted cereal. It "improved" my mood and made me physically more active while it simultaneously made me spacey with reduced stamina. I was addicted to the sugar rush. I would forgo eating the vital nutrient-rich, natural foods necessary for optimal development, function, and repair. In addition to changing my brain chemistry, the excess sugar changed my intestinal environment from what it would be if I had eaten natural foods to an environment that favored overgrowth of troublesome microorganisms. I had intestinal discomfort and allergies and had trouble concentrating. As I outgrew sugar-frosted cereals, I was indoctrinated with corn– or cane–sugar-rich soft drinks as part of the new "generation."

Recently, Big Tobacco (BT) has been successfully

sued numerous times for big bucks for knowingly endangering and impairing consumers' health while addicting them to their products.

Today, obesity is overtaking tobacco as the number-one public-health hazard. The rise in obesity is associated with consumption of commercially refined foods, particularly sugars, in unprecedented quantities. We crave sugar to give us quick fixes of mental or physical energy in order to overcome our deficiencies in diet, rest, and exercise. We store away much of the excess calories of the sugar fix as fat. Should Big Sugar (BS) also answer for knowingly promoting ill health and premature demise of its consumers? Should promotion of sugar-laden health-robbing foods be banned on cartoons and other kids' television shows? How much more BS can we stand?

Lifestyles have changed irrevocably for most of us. We are unlikely to forgo our habituated use of convenience foods and refrigerators to go back to nature to forage for wildly grown nutrition in the woods. We are unlikely to eliminate the habituated joys of sweetened food for less tasty alternatives. We have choices. We can include more natural organically grown whole foods in our diets and take nutritional supplements. We can use nontoxic substitutes for corn- and cane-derived sweeteners. One such substitute is Xylitol. Xylitol is naturally occurring and has additional health benefits beyond that of simply replacing sucrose and fructose sugars.

The Sweet Miracle of Xylitol is best told by one of the world's foremost public communicators and scientific experts on Xylitol, Fran Gare, N.D., M.S. Although Xylitol has been in use for quite a while, it has never been used to its greatest potential. Until recently, the technology was lacking to make Xylitol economically practical, and qualified communicators were unavailable to tell the world how to take advantage of what it has to offer. Fortunately, both are now available. With our health under siege from sugar-related diseases, this availability could hardly be more timely.

Thank you, Dr. Gare, for bringing the Xylitol story to light. Thank you for your many years of relentless dedication to nutritional research and developing ways to make the world a healthier place.

—Martin Dayton,
D.O., M.D., F.A.A.F.P.

Preface

I s Xylitol a sweet miracle? Yes! In my sixty-two years of living (half of which I have spent as a health practitioner), I have not experienced too many miraculous happenings. But there was that Saturday afternoon a few years back when I attended a medical seminar.

As I was leaving the meeting, I saw a booth outside advertising all-natural, sugar-free gums and mints. I've always believed that sugar-free is the way to live and have tried every sugar substitute imaginable, from those that tasted fine but were laden with chemicals to those that were all-natural but make you cringe upon contact with your tongue. I didn't expect much from this new product, but I felt obligated to give it a go and reluctantly walked over to the booth.

During my years as director of nutrition of The Atkins Center for Clinical Nutrition and in private practice, I have treated thousands of patients who wanted to lose weight (many of whom had diabetes). Giving up sugar was a personal anguish for almost every patient, and it saddened me that I could not healthfully and "tastefully" satisfy their sweet cravings. In a way, it had become a life's dream to find a sweet substance that was free of chemicals, healthful, and looked and tasted just like sugar.

And then the "sweet miracle" happened. The sweetener used in the gums and mints at the booth was an all-natural substance called Xylitol (*xyl* is Greek for "wood")—a sugar substitute from Finland originally made from the bark of birch trees. And I learned it had been approved by the FDA as a food additive for more than twenty-five years!

My first surprise was that Xylitol looked exactly like sugar. My excitement grew when I tasted it. While I knew that this was not sugar, my taste buds were convinced that it was. Believe it or not, the best was still to come. There was an aftertaste that lasted about ten minutes—the aftertaste was *the sweetness of sugar!*

I know that I sound like a runaway advertisement for Xylitol, and the truth is that I extol its praises whenever I can. When you begin to use Xylitol as your sweetener, it will change your life. That is why I am writing this book. I want you and your family to enjoy the sweet miracle of decadently delicious treats that can help you become healthier, thinner, and virtually younger as you enjoy eating them.

Introduction

The evidence is undeniable: Sugar can make you overweight and sick. The latest research and media reports show that diets high in sugar and refined carbohydrates make us fat and unhealthy!

"What if Fat Doesn't Make You Fat? What if It's All Been a Big Fat Lie?" These provoking words graced the cover of the *New York Times Magazine* on July 7, 2002. The article examined the current American Diabetes Association (ADA) Pyramid and the American diet and reached a very specific conclusion: the low-fat, high-carbohydrate, high-sugar diet of most Americans is causing obesity and disease.

A recent ABC News report that featured an interview with Dr. Walter Willett, Chairman of the Department of Nutrition at Harvard University, also brought to light some serious questions about our diet and nutrition. In particular, it focused on the USDA Pyramid, which was designed by the government and is supposedly one of the most trustworthy guides for nutrition. "The dietary pyramid was out of date the day it was printed, but it's even more out of date given the evidence that's accrued since that time," claimed Willett. "We have good evidence now that the high intake of refined starches and sugars will increase risk of diabetes and heart disease," he added.

A separate piece on the low-fat myth by *20/20*, which also ran recently, echoes Willett's sentiments. In that piece, Dr. Timothy Johnson, the medical editor at ABC News, states, "The theory was that a low-fat/high-carb diet would control weight and help prevent killer diseases. But most of the studies that followed actually failed to show a direct link between fat in the diet and heart disease and cancer. But by then it was too late—even science couldn't shake the prevailing wisdom that all fats are bad, and all carbs are good." Dr. Johnson concludes that "there's plenty of compelling evidence to do the following. Get rid of the refined starches and sugars . . . eat more vegetables and fruit, eat lean protein and healthy fats. You'll lose weight and feel better and may reduce your risk for heart disease."

The theme of these recent media reports is an obvious but compelling one. The diet many of us practice and have always believed to be healthy—low-fat, high-carb—is, in fact, anything but healthy. The percentage of Americans who are considered obese seems to grow every year. In fact, the incidence of obesity is projected to grow by almost 14 percent by 2010. And what's most troubling is that a large part of that growth is expected to be in children and adolescents. In addition, heart disease, diabetes, and a host of other diseases are on the rise. Again, what's probably most disturbing is that our children are being affected. The diabetes epidemic has expanded to include adolescents. Before the low-fat diet fad, we saw very few cases of type II (adult-onset) diabetes in children. Today, it is a rapidly expanding disease in the adolescent group.

We know that our current diet is compromising our health and the health of our children. But what do we do about it? We're so used to eating certain foods, foods we've grown to love, that it's difficult to change our diets entirely all at once. So maybe it's unrealistic to expect people in one day to go from a low-fat, high-carb, high-sugar diet to the healthier diet that Dr. Johnson recommends above: eating more vegetables and fruit, lean protein, and healthy fats, and getting rid of the starches and sugars. Changing our diets and making ourselves healthier may need to be accomplished in steps.

This book is about taking one of those steps: eliminating refined sugar from our diets. Seems like a scary proposition, right? Almost all of us love sweet things—cakes, cookies, ice cream, or whatever it may be. It's almost always a welcome vice. But after you've learned how damaging sugar can be and you are introduced to the sugar alternative that tastes just like sugar (but promotes health rather than destroys it), you won't think twice about taking this huge step.

THE SUGAR PROBLEM

Sugar has been a part of our diet for centuries. However, the troubling thing is that Americans today are consuming sugar in higher quantities than ever before. In fact, sugar consumption is so high in this country that the Center for Science in the Public Interest (CSPI) petitioned the FDA to set a maximum recommended daily intake (Daily Value) for added sugars and to require labels to disclose the percentage of the Daily Value a food provides.

This "sugar problem" can also be linked to the predominance of the low-fat diet in our culture. As low-fat manufacturers reduce the fats in foods, they add chemicals and loads of sugars to make the foods taste "good." So even if you don't realize that your low-fat diet is high in sugar, chances are it is. But why is sugar so bad?

Some of the Bodily Harm Moderate-to High-Sugar Diets Can Cause

When you ingest simple sugar (table sugar, or sucrose), it begins digesting in your mouth. Your body sends a message to your pancreas that sugar is on its way, and your pancreas begins to excrete insulin to help the cells absorb sugar so your body can use it.

When you eat too much sugar, your pancreas makes too much insulin and your cells can't absorb all of it. When this happens, the insulin remains in your bloodstream. That is when health problems begin.

The following is a list of the major health problems that eating a diet moderately high or high in sugar can cause:

- Hormone-related cancers. High insulin levels raise the amount of the estrogen hormones (especially estrone) in the blood.

- Hypoglycemia, which can lead to diabetes, which, in

For a list of sixty-seven (footnoted) ways that sugar can harm your body, you can visit www.nancyappleton.com, the website of Nancy Appleton, Ph.D., author of *Lick the Sugar Habit*, an influential book about the dangers of sugar.

turn, can lead to diminished eyesight (even blindness) and amputation of limbs.

- Autoimmune/immune-deficiency disorders like arthritis, allergies, and asthma.

- A mineral imbalance in your body, which can lead to conditions such as osteoporosis.

- Elevated triglycerides and elevated levels of "bad" cholesterol (low-density lipoproteins, or LDLs), which can lead to heart disease.

- Tooth decay and periodontal disease, which can lead to heart disease.

- Learning dysfunctions, forgetfulness, and possibly senility (even Alzheimer's disease).

- Obesity—an epidemic that we are trying to eat our way out of.

ARE WE BEGINNING TO SEE THE LIGHT?

While statistics show that obesity, heart disease, and diabetes are on the rise in this country, there is some hope.

Tides have begun to shift from low-fat (high-sugar) diets to high-protein, moderate–healthy-fat, low-carbohydrate (no refined sugar) diets. And the United States has a share of more than one-third of the market for functional foods, those foods that function to improve our health.

Late in 2001, for the first time, functional foods became the most covered nutraceutical media topic. Leading the functional food market are consumers who know that the low-fat/high-carbohydrate diet has caused an epidemic of diabetes, heart disease, hypertension, digestive disorders, and immune-depressive diseases. Shoppers are growing more concerned about their health and the health of their families. Consequently, they are supporting breakthroughs in sweet goods, looking to sugar alternatives to satisfy their sweet tooth.

Consumers are supporting the breakthrough technologies in "sweet goods" designed for:

- Carbohydrate restriction and control.

- Diet/weight loss.

- Diabetes.

- Bowel and digestive disorders.

- Heart disease.

- Rapid aging.

According to Food Marketing Institute/Prevention's 2000 "Self-Care" Survey, 75 percent of supermarket shoppers purchased foods to lower the risk of developing a condition or illness (up from 54 percent in 1998). For the first time, about half said that wanting to slow the aging process influenced their grocery purchases. In addition, consumers say they've used various types of diets to lose or maintain weight: 63 percent by controlling sugar intake and 49 percent by eating fewer carbohydrates.

GOOD NEWS, BUT . . .

The good news is that the necessity for dietary changes has finally begun to resound in the minds of many Americans. But there's still plenty of room for improvement—and not just on the part of consumers.

The functional food industry is very much a work in progress. Manufacturers of sugar-free products and sugar alternatives have no shortage of products on the market, but as you will soon discover, most of these products are far from ideal. Some may cause more long-term health problems than they solve, others cause unpleasant side effects, and still others just taste awful.

I previously mentioned Dr. Nancy Appleton, the author of *Lick the Sugar Habit* and other books about the dangers of eating sugar. Nancy told me that she is a purist. She believes that everyone should stop eating sugar NOW! She thinks sugar is so bad that she is currently doing an infomercial for a sugar-free gum. Nancy told me that nutritionists think that the gum is a great idea, but they won't use it because it is made with chemicals.

So it seems that consumers like us will have to make do until researchers can find that ideal product—one that prevents the long-term health problems that sugar causes, has no unpleasant side effects, tastes just like sugar, and is all natural. Or will we?

WE'VE HAD THE ANSWER ALL ALONG

For the past twenty-five years, consumers in Finland, Russia, China, and a host of other countries have been using a product that meets all of the above criteria. But for one reason or another, it hadn't made its way into the American marketplace. Manufacturers' labs are filled with scientists trying to concoct the ideal sugar alternative. And all this time, all they had to do was look across the Atlantic or the Pacific for the answer.

This seemingly ideal product is finally being realized by American manufacturers and is slowly entering the marketplace in this country. It could potentially improve the health of millions while allowing us to continue to eat those sweet foods that we've grown to love. It is all natural and tastes just like sugar, and has been proven to prevent diabetes, help with weight loss, and improve dental health. This "sweet miracle," of course, is Xylitol.

1.

The Sweetener of Choice

Why is it important to know about Xylitol, the all-natural, healthy sweetener? Because your health and the health of your children and grandchildren are at stake!

A survey conducted by the Gallup Organization for the Calorie Control Council found that as many as 90 percent of adult Americans—173 million people—eat sugar-free and other diet foods on a daily basis. The astounding part of this is that there has been a 28 percent increase in these numbers over the last three years. And those numbers are rising!

I have found that when the public listens, it is a healthy sign, but when people unequivocally trust what they hear without thinking it through, wrong choices are frequently made. This is often the case when we are choosing "diet foods." Up until recently, "diet foods" were low-fat, high-sugar foods (like 300-calorie low-fat diet muffins). Current studies have shown that these foods actually cause people to gain weight and increase their bodies' vulnerability to diabetes, heart disease, and even cancer.

Our concept of diet, weight loss, and health has

changed. Foods low in refined carbohydrates (like sugar, white flour, pasta, and white rice) are becoming the foods to avoid eating. Sugar-free foods are the new diet foods. This chapter is designed to help you make more intelligent sugar-free choices.

My ideas about sugar substitutes were developed over the years as I struggled to bake great-tasting recipes for the sugar-free cookbooks I wrote with Dr. Atkins. At that time, I only had artificial sugar substitutes to work with. There are now 35 million people who eat these on a daily basis. To understand why they do, think about this: Imagine that you are eating a rich, delicious chocolate fudge brownie or a bowl of ice cream topped with a chocolate chip biscotti. How does it make you feel? Do you feel guilty? Do you feel like you are doing an "evil deed" to your body?

Well, you never again have to feel guilty about eating dessert. Truly! Even if you have diabetes, hypoglycemia, or sugar allergies, or if you are simply health conscious and don't wish to eat sugar, you can enjoy sweet foods when you use Xylitol as your sweetener.

WHAT IS XYLITOL?

Xylitol is an all-natural substance that is produced by your body during normal glucose metabolism. Xylitol is found in nature in berries, mushrooms, lettuce, hard woods, and corncobs. It looks and tastes like sugar but with fewer calories and carbohydrates, and teaspoon for teaspoon behaves like sugar in most of your recipes (however, it will not caramelize).

There isn't another sugar alternative that offers this much. And, if you care about your health, consider this:

- Xylitol does not cause an insulin reaction in the body, making it desirable for people with diabetes and hypoglycemia and for low-carb dieters.

- Xylitol rates a 7 on the glycemic index, a ranking of foods based on their immediate effect on blood glucose (blood sugar) levels. The glycemic index rates foods on a scale of 1–100; foods with the lowest numbers are the healthiest. (Table sugar, or sucrose, rates a 110; glucose rates a 100.)

- Xylitol helps prevent tooth decay.

- Xylitol reduces plaque formation on teeth.

- Xylitol increases salivary flow to aid in the repair of damaged tooth enamel.

- Xylitol may help prevent osteoporosis.

- Xylitol stops the development of strep bacteria in the mouth and intestines.

- Xylitol has 40 percent fewer calories than sugar and is as sweet as sugar.

- Xylitol has 75 percent fewer carbohydrates than sugar.

- Xylitol has been the subject of more than 1,500 research studies.

THE EVOLUTION OF XYLITOL

Xylitol has been known to the world of organic chemistry

for more than 100 years. It was first made by German and French chemists in 1890. Humans and animals have eaten it during their entire evolution because it occurs naturally in berries (especially raspberries), plums, cauliflower, lettuce, and many other plants.

By 1930, Xylitol had been purified, but it was not until after World War II that the sugar shortage in countries like Finland forced researchers to look at alternative sweeteners. At that time, the interest in Xylitol became strong enough for it to be stabilized so that it would not break down when used in foods. Folklore relates that during the time the Fins were eating Xylitol instead of sugar, the nation became healthier. In fact, it was during this period that researchers began to realize Xylitol's insulin-independent nature (it metabolizes in your body without the use of insulin).

In 1975, a Finnish company began the first large-scale production of Xylitol. A year later, this company was joined by the Swiss company F. Hoffman La-Roche, and together they founded Xyrofin. Xyrofin is currently owned by the Finnish Sugar Company, which has merged with Cultor International.

Still, we in America had not heard of Xylitol because we had an abundant amount of sugar available to us. But about the same time that Finland began to manufacture Xylitol, other countries—the former Soviet Union, Japan, Germany, and Italy—were producing it for use in their domestic markets. In Japan, it was being used, among other things, as an IV infusion to resuscitate patients from diabetic comas.

Xylitol first arrived on the American market in 1975

in the form of chewing gum. I remember our dentist giving the gum to my children. But it did not catch on here as it did in other countries. Leaf, a Finnish company, has been making gums, mints, candies, and toothpaste using Xylitol as the sweetener for years. Up until now, we have been importing those healthy treats. In the U.S. today, Xylitol is sold under the brand names Perfect Sweet, Miracle Sweet, and Healthy Sweet. Yet I'm sure most of you don't even recognize the names of these products.

Expense has thus far been the problem with Xylitol. It was and still is far more expensive than sugar, the substance it healthfully replaces. However, The Sweet Life, Inc., a Miami corporation, now buys Xylitol in volume and has been able to bring down its price low enough to market it in patented, made-in-America sugar-free and grain-free cake mixes. The all-natural mixes, available in chocolate, almond, and maple pecan flavors, use Xylitol as the only sweetener. (See Appendix: Xylitol Products.) The sweets—brownies, muffins, cookies, candies, ice creams, and puddings—made from these mixes taste just like (or even better than) the "real thing." I feel certain that this is only the beginning of Xylitol-sweetened products.

HOW XYLITOL IS MADE

Originally, Xylitol was extracted from birch or beech wood chips, and in some places, it is still made that way. Hemicellulose (the scientific name for Xylitol) is a *xylan*, a long polysaccharide molecule consisting of D-xylose units. Xylans are present in birch and beech and are also present in rice, wheat, and cottonseed hulls; in sugar-cane husks; and in corncobs and stalks.

Since corncobs are a major waste product of the food industry and are easily available in large quantities, most Xylitol is manufactured from them. India is developing an industry making Xylitol from sugar-cane husks (a process that began in Taiwan). If the process is successful, the cost of Xylitol could be lowered worldwide.

In the most economical of the manufacturing processes, xylan molecules are first hydrolyzed into D-xylose, which is reduced to Xylitol. Another manufacturing process involves fermenting corncobs, but it is a much more expensive method and therefore is not often used.

THE CHEMICAL PROFILE OF XYLITOL

Remember, Xylitol is a natural product; it is produced from natural sources—birch bark, blueberry skins, corncobs, and other substances that occur in nature. What is interesting is that the final product—Xylitol—looks like sugar, is as sweet as sugar, but has a chemical profile that is different from sugar.

The Xylitol molecule contains five carbons and five hydroxyl groups. This makes it a sugar alcohol of the pentol type. Five-carbon sugar alcohols are antimicrobial—they do not support the growth of bacteria. Xylitol actually destroys streptococci and other bacteria, both in the mouth and in the intestines. Six-carbon sugars and sugar alcohols like sucrose (table sugar), however, support the growth of streptococci and other bacteria.

OTHER DIFFERENCES BETWEEN XYLITOL AND SUGAR

The way that Xylitol is metabolized makes it different from sugar and even different from other sugar alcohols (such as sorbitol). As previously mentioned, Xylitol is a natural product that regularly occurs in the glucose metabolism of humans, other animals, and some plants. Dietary Xylitol is easily metabolized and does not raise insulin levels. About one-third of the Xylitol you eat is absorbed by your liver; the other two-thirds travels to your intestines where it is broken down by gut bacteria into short-chain fatty acids that are utilized by the body (mostly in the liver).

The Physical and Chemical Properties of Xylitol

Molecular Weight: 152.15

Appearance: White, crystalline powder

Odor: None

PH in water (1 g/10 ml): 5 to 7

Boiling Point: 126°C (at 760 mm)

Melting Point: 92° to 96°C

Solubility at 20°C: 169 g in 100 g of water, sparingly/soluble in ethanol and methanol

Heat of Solution: −34.8 cal/g (endothermic)

Calorific Value: 2.4 calories per gram

OTHER SUGAR ALTERNATIVES (AND WHY THEY CAN'T COMPARE)

Other Sugar Alcohols—Polyols

Scientists call polyols "sugar alcohols" because part of their structures chemically resemble sugar and part of their structures resemble alcohol. However, they are neither sugars nor alcohols.

Sugar alcohols are digested more slowly than sugar, affecting insulin levels less dramatically. Actually, little or no insulin is needed to metabolize them. Xylitol is a polyol, but I am convinced that the other polyols do not measure up.

Xylitol prevents tooth decay; while some of the sugar alcohols may not promote tooth decay, they certainly don't prevent it. In addition, the side effect of diarrhea is not the problem for Xylitol that it is for other sugar alcohols. When eaten in excess, sugar alcohols have a laxative effect. This is because the body cannot completely digest them. Eating more than 60 grams of Xylitol may cause slight cramping and mild diarrhea during the first few days that you eat it. But Xylitol is made by the body, and the body has enzymes to break it down. In a short time, your enzymes go to work and the laxative effect subsides.

In one study, 200 grams a day of Xylitol was consumed without incidence of diarrhea, but I wouldn't push it that far. I suggest 50–70 grams spread throughout the day. That's a healthy amount, even for people with diabetes and hypoglycemia.

Other sugar alcohols do not have brand names. This

is because they are not available in supermarkets or specialty markets. They are available in food laboratories and manufacturing plants where they are added to sugar-free foods to make them taste sweeter.

Most Commonly Used Polyols

Sorbitol, the most widely used polyol, is about 60 percent as sweet as sugar. It is a six-carbon sugar alcohol (one that doesn't prevent tooth decay), and because it ferments, it is likely to cause diarrhea, even when eaten in small amounts. Sorbitol occurs in a wide variety of fruits and berries. However, it is produced commercially by the hydrogenation of glucose.

Maltitol is about 90 percent as sweet as sugar and is the newly favored sweetener for sugar-free chocolates because it gives foods a creamy texture. It is made by the hydrogenation of maltose, which is obtained from starch. It does not raise insulin or blood glucose levels, so it is safe for people with diabetes and is good to use on low-carbohydrate diets. Consumption of more than 15 grams at one time can lead to stomach cramps and diarrhea.

Mannitol is 70 percent as sweet as sugar. It occurs naturally in beets, celery, and olives. Commercially, it is made from hydrogen and glucose (corn sugar). It is used with other sweeteners in many sugar-free foods, but like sorbitol, it must be eaten in small amounts to avoid stomach cramps and diarrhea.

Lactitol, derived from lactose, is the least sweet (one-third as sweet as sugar) and lowest in calories (2 calories per gram) of these sweeteners. It works well when combined with other sugar alcohols in candies and ice cream. For instance, it prevents ice cream from becoming frosty.

Other Natural Sugar Alternatives

This category of sweeteners is not a group of sugar alcohols. These sweeteners come from natural sources.

Stevia is an all-natural herb that the Food and Drug Administration (FDA) insists is an "unsafe food additive." Studies, however, reveal that stevia has been used by millions of people around the world, and there has never been an ill effect attributed to it. If you would like to see the studies done on the safety and healing benefits of stevia and the great lengths to which the FDA has gone in an effort to keep this naturally sweet herb out of foods you eat, you can visit www.stevia.net/bookburning.htm.

Stevia is 300 times sweeter than sugar but does not contain calories or carbohydrates. It does leave a strong licorice aftertaste. If you don't mind the licorice aftertaste, you can buy stevia in a health food store (it is approved as an herb) and add it to your foods. It is heat stable so it retains its flavor when used in cooking.

Fructose and high fructose corn syrup have been presented to the public as natural sweeteners. After all, fructose is fruit sugar, and what could be better or more natural? Well that was what fructose was twenty years ago, but not today. Today, fructose is not made from fruit. It is a commercially refined sugar made from corn. The fructose of today is lacking most of the health benefits of the fructose that came from fruit. High fructose corn syrup is known to cause elevated cholesterol and triglyceride levels. The FDA claims not to have done any studies on the safety of fructose.

Non-Nutritive Artificial Sweeteners

The following sugar substitutes are made in laboratories. They are widely used chemical sweetening agents.

Aspartame is probably the most widely used of the sugar substitutes. It is also the substance that the FDA receives more complaints about on a daily basis than any other food chemical. Aspartame, better known as NutraSweet, is a combination of two amino acids (protein components)—L-aspartic acid and L-phenylalanine. It is about 180 times sweeter than table sugar (sucrose). The FDA approved aspartame in 1981 (after years of not approving it) as a tabletop sweetener. It was the first low-calorie sweetener approved by the FDA in more than twenty-five years. The FDA claims that more than 100 studies on the toxic effects of aspartame as well as the clinical studies it has reviewed confirm that aspartame is safe for the general public. Consumption of aspartame can result in the production of methanol, formaldehyde, and formate—substances that can be toxic at high doses. In fact, H. J. Roberta, M.D., reports, "Well before aspartame was approved of as safe, research reports began being published about aspartame causing neurological damage (mostly because of an accumulation of formaldehyde in the brain and nervous system)."

I remember hearing about these negative side effects in 1995 when I was director of nutrition of The Atkins Center for Clinical Nutrition. As a result of these reports, I stopped recommending aspartame to patients. Since I had not yet been introduced to Xylitol, I asked patients to switch to the natural sweetener stevia discussed previously or to choose another of the approved sweeteners on the market. Almost immediately, patients began to report that their memory improved, they could concentrate for longer periods of time, and they had fewer headaches.

For more information on the dangers of aspartame, you can read Dr. Roberta's well-researched books, *Sweet-'Ner Dearest, Bittersweet Vignettes About Aspartame (NutraSweet)* (Sunshine Sentinel Press, 1992) and *Aspartame Disease: An Ignored Epidemic* (Sunshine Sentinel Press, 2001).

Acesulfame-K (*acesulfame potassium*) is 200 times sweeter than sugar and has no caloric value. It is marketed under the names Sunett and The Sweet One. I find this sweetener intensely sweet when I cook with it. In tea and coffee, I find that it has a chemical aftertaste.

The fifteen volumes of research presented to the FDA by the American Hoechst Corporation, manufacturer of acesulfame-K, claimed that acesulfame-K is not metabolized by the body. However, six months before the sweetener was approved in 1988, the Center for Science in the Public Interest (CSPI), a Washington, D.C.–based consumer group, sent a warning to the FDA saying that animals fed acesulfame-K in two different studies developed more tumors than those that did not receive the compound. The details are reported by Ruth Winter in her book *A Consumer's Dictionary of Food Additives* (Three Rivers Press, 1999). An FDA press release stated that it had considered CSPI's concerns and concluded that "any tumors found were typical of what could routinely be expected and were not due to feeding Acesulfame-K." In another study cited by CSPI, diabetic rats had a higher blood level of cholesterol when fed the sweetener.

Most scientists reacted to the findings by the CSPI in a similar manner. They agreed that the tests were incomplete and flawed, and that more testing was needed. Lorenzo Tomatis, former director of the International Agency for Research on Cancer, stated, "There are several serious flaws in the design and conduct of the tests. The only conclusion one can draw from looking at the available results is that *Acesulfame K* should be tested in a proper way before an evaluation of its carcinogenicity can be made."

Saccharin has been in use since 1879. It is 300 times sweeter than sugar. It is marketed under trade names such as Sweet'N Low. Saccharin was a GRAS (generally recognized as safe) substance when Congress passed the Food Additives Amendment to the Food, Drug and Cosmetics Act. This amendment required premarket approval from the FDA for food additives developed before 1958. Despite concerns that saccharin was linked to cancer in lab animals, it did receive approval and is still GRAS.

Saccharin is, in fact, the most studied of all of the non-nutritive, artificial sweeteners. More than 2,300 studies have been conducted; many done in the early 1900s indicated that saccharin is a carcinogen. Of note was a Canadian study that almost had saccharin banned from the U.S. marketplace. It showed conclusively that saccharin caused bladder cancer in rats. Following the Canadian study, there were media reports that the rats that had developed bladder cancers had been fed the equivalent of 800 diet sodas per day. The average person using saccharin eats less than one ounce of the sweetener a year. (See the inset "The Public Wanted Saccharin" on page 23.)

Sucralose is the newest non-nutritive sweetener. It is 600 times sweeter than sugar, yet it is derived from sugar. A white crystalline powder that tastes a lot like sugar, it is more intense in its sweetness. I have noticed a burning sensation in my mouth when I eat foods made with sucralose.

The manufacture of sucralose involves a multistep patented manufacturing process. Three atoms of chlorine are substituted for three hydroxl (hydrogen) groups on the sugar molecule. The manufacturer says that this process renders the sugar indigestible and calorie-free. *Sucralose* is bulked-up with maltodexrine, a starchy powder, so it will measure more like sugar and is marketed under the trade name Splenda.

There have been only nineteen research studies on sucralose, but they speak volumes. Research in animals has shown that sucralose can cause many problems in rodents. The following are some of the problems found in the studies:

The Public Wanted Saccharin

The public cried out; more studies were needed on saccharin. The "Saccharin Study and Labeling Act" was passed, placing a two-year moratorium on banning saccharin. Saccharin remained on the market. However, it did wear a label that read: "Use of this product may be hazardous to your health."

Thirty extensive research studies on humans indicated no association between saccharin and cancer. One researcher, Dr. Samuel Cohen, professor and chairman of the Department of Pathology and Microbiology at the University of Nebraska Medical Center, has performed studies in which he fed high doses of a sodium salt, including sodium ascorbate (vitamin C) and sodium saccharin, to male rats to alter the rat urine. This may lead to the formation of a substance that may lead to the formation of tumors in rats' bladders. Dr. Cohen found that the sodium salts produced tumors only when administered at high doses and only in rats. (He also performed the tests on monkeys.) Therefore, he concluded, the mechanism by which the rats develop cancer is specific to rats. "The lack of effect in mice, and more importantly in monkeys, combined with the strong epidemiological evidence from humans and our understanding of mechanism, strongly support the conclusion that exposure to saccharin does not pose a carcinogenic risk to humans," Dr. Cohen stated in a paper.

In December 2000, President Clinton signed a bill removing the warning label from saccharin-sweetened products.

- Shrunken thymus glands (up to 40 percent shrinkage).

- Enlarged liver and kidneys.

- Atrophy of lymph follicles in the spleen and thymus.

- Reduced growth rate.

- Decreased red blood cell count.

- Inflammation of the pelvis.

- Extension of the pregnancy period.

- Aborted pregnancy.

- Decreased fetal body weights and placental weights.

- Diarrhea.

Despite the manufacturer's claims to the contrary, sucralose is significantly absorbed and metabolized by the body. According to the FDA's "Final Rule" report, 11 to 27 percent of sucralose is absorbed in humans, and the rest is excreted unchanged in feces. According to the Japanese Food Sanitation Council, as much as 40 percent of ingested sucralose is absorbed.

About 20 to 30 percent of absorbed sucralose is metabolized. Both the metabolites and unchanged absorbed sucralose are excreted in urine. The absorbed sucralose has been found to concentrate in the liver, kidneys, and gastrointestinal tract. According to The Sucralose Toxicity Information Center, sucralose is broken down "into small amounts of 1,6-dichlorofructose, a chemical which has not been adequately tested in humans." There seem to be many more questions surrounding sucralose—questions of purity and of pesticide and heavy metal contamination.

Those who defend the use of sucralose quote the FDA papers reporting the animal studies done on Splenda, the brand name of sucralose. Like the saccharin studies, they were done using huge doses (the equivalent of a 150-pound person eating 17,500 teaspoons a day). This sounds like a reasonable objection, and I could feel comfortable with it if we were not absorbing sucralose. Absorbed, it can accumulate in your body over a period of time. This fact, plus the lack of long-term human studies (there have been only ninety-three short-term animal studies on sucralose) and the fact that sucralose has not yet been approved for use in Europe, gives me an uneasy feeling about it.

In addition, Whole Foods Market, a food market that sells only all natural and organic foods, has placed sucralose on the list of substances not allowed in its stores. That alone is enough to keep me from recommending it. Thinking sucralose was safe, on the advice of my food technologist, I originally had used it in my *Fran Gare's Decadent Desserts* products, and have since removed it. The desserts taste even better without it. There was a slight bitterness that is gone.

To find out more about the toxic side of sucralose, visit the Sucralose Toxicity Center at:

http://www.holisticmed.com/splenda/ *or*
http://mercola.com/2000/dec/3/.

2.

The Healing Effects of Xylitol

Imagine being able to indulge yourself with cake, candy, and ice cream and grow healthier all the while. What a notion! It's a notion that becomes real when you choose to eat foods sweetened with Xylitol. Consider these numbers:

- 17 million Americans suffer from some form of diabetes.

- 10 million Americans are estimated to suffer from osteo-porosis and almost 34 million more are estimated to have low bone mass, placing them at increased risk for osteoporosis.

- 50 percent of Americans suffer from moderate to severe tooth decay.

- 25 percent of women have *Candida albicans* (yeast infection) present in their system.

Xylitol not only helps in the prevention and treatment of all of these diseases, but it has a number of other sig-nificant health-promoting properties. In this chapter, we will explore how sugar-laden diets can leave our bodies compromised and disease-ridden, and how Xylitol, more than any other sugar alternative, can restore our health and vitality.

INSULIN-RESISTANT DISORDERS: DIABETES AND SYNDROME X

Insulin-resistant related disorders (diabetes and hypoglycemia) affect the health of about 19 million Americans (10 million diagnosed and about 9 million undiagnosed). It has reached epidemic proportions in this country, so much so that doctors are considering testing patients for pre-diabetes. Why? Because insulin-resistant disorders are dangerous, and they can lead to the three deadliest diseases we know—diabetes, hypertension/heart disease, and cancer.

It All Begins with Insulin Resistance

When you eat a starchy or sugary food, it begins to digest in your mouth. The digestive enzyme amylase breaks down sugar and other simple carbohydrates into glucose (blood sugar). Your pancreas gets the message that sugar is on the way, and it secretes the hormone insulin as a way of regulating the amount of sugar in your body. Your body uses blood insulin to transport glucose from your blood to target muscle cells where it can be stored and used for energy.

If your diet consists of only a small amount of simple carbohydrates (sugar, fruit, white flours, and some starchy vegetables), the insulin works to regulate the sugars, and then it is taken into your cells as energy. All is well.

However, when you continually eat a diet high in simple carbohydrates, your pancreas is constantly producing insulin, so much so that the target cells in your muscles do not respond well to the amounts of insulin in your bloodstream. The cells do not take the insulin in. Your pancreas gets the message that your cells need insulin and it makes more insulin. Instead of being taken up by the cells, the glucose and insulin remain in your bloodstream, causing degenerative problems in your body.

Glucose in your bloodstream (which travels to every cell in your body) is a major source of dangerous free radicals that break down, rather than build up, cells. A free radical is an electron that has lost its mate. While seeking a new mate, the free radical travels in the body, attacking healthy cells and breaking them apart. Free-radical damage is the cause of all degenerative diseases, including cancer.

Diabetes: Types I and II

When glucose levels rise in the blood and the glucose is not used by the body, type II diabetes results. Diabetes is essentially high blood sugar (fasting levels above 120 mg/dL).

Type I diabetes is a genetic disease in which the body does not make insulin; it occurs at birth or in early childhood. Type II diabetes, a condition in which the body does not properly use insulin, may have a genetic component, but today it is more often than not carbohydrate-induced. Because of the great amounts of simple carbohydrates in the American diet (mostly carbohydrates and fats), we see type II diabetes beginning in young adults. According to The American Diabetes Association, between 90 and 95 percent of all people with diabetes over the age of twenty have type II diabetes.

Diabetes Leads to Heart Disease: Syndrome X

Syndrome X was named about ten years ago. It refers to a condition characterized by high fasting glucose levels (above 120 mg/dL) and elevated triglycerides and cholesterol levels (especially LDL cholesterol levels). Research indicates that death from heart disease follows a U-shaped curve based on insulin levels. The higher the insulin levels, the greater the chance of developing heart disease.

The following study reported in *The Journal of the American Medical Association* in 1998 is often quoted. The study looked at traditional risk factors compared to fasting insulin levels in individuals who had no trace of heart disease. Researchers wanted to see which were more predictive of developing heart disease over a five-year period. The study found that fasting insulin levels are more than twice as predictive of the development of heart disease as LDL cholesterol, which is currently considered the gold standard. The second most predictive factor is elevated triglycerides—the first sign of *hyperinsulinemia* (too much insulin in the blood). The HDL/ triglyceride ratio is just behind elevated insulin levels as a risk factor—again a surrogate marker for testing for hyperinsulinemia.

Dietary Fats and Hyperinsulinemia

In the past, it was believed that eating fat was the cause of high cholesterol. Today, we know that it is the carbohydrates that are eaten with the fat that cause most of the problems. It is true that when you eat more fat, cholesterol levels go up, but that is usually because you eat more carbohydrates with the fat. It is true that fat is the raw material from which cholesterol is made, but insulin runs the cellular machinery that actually manufactures cholesterol. If you stop eating carbohydrates and your insulin levels go down, your cells will not be able to convert dietary fat to cholesterol.

Hypertension

Study after study has revealed an unusually high incidence of hypertension in people who have elevated glucose and insulin levels. Especially when the people are overweight.

Experiments have been conducted to lower insulin levels in hypertensive patients. In almost all of the cases, lowering insulin levels in these patients also lowered their blood pressure. On the other hand, experiments that just lowered blood pressure did not lower insulin levels.

The researchers have found that insulin may not only cause hypertension, but also may promote hypertensive complications and other cardiovascular diseases. These studies were reported by L. Landsberg in the *Journal of Clinical and Experimental Hypertension* in 1996.

Insulin and Fertility

John E. Nestler, M.D., authored an interesting and worthwhile article on the website of the American Diabetes Association. Dr. Nestler reports that a disorder in women of reproductive age, known as polycystic ovary syndrome (PCOS), frequently features insulin resistance. The result of insulin resistance in these women is an increase in free testosterone. (Free testosterone is testosterone that is available for the body to use as opposed to bound testosterone, which is not free to be used by the body.) Testosterone opposes estrogen in the body. An increase in free testosterone can cause infertility.

Xylitol's Insulin Connection

- Xylitol does not raise insulin levels and does not raise cholesterol levels. It is safe for people with diabetes and people with high cholesterol and triglyceride levels.

- Xylitol ranks as a 7 on the glycemic index, indicating that it requires only tiny amounts of insulin to be completely metabolized.

- Xylitol assists insulin in getting into the target muscle cells.

- Xylitol is low in calories.

- Xylitol has a slow, steady energy release.

- Xylitol will keep your body from going into ketosis (abnormal levels of ketones in the body) because it helps the body to use fats and to balance insulin levels.

- Xylitol reduces carbohydrate cravings and helps curb binge eating.

OSTEOPOROSIS

Osteoporosis is a major health problem for 44 million Americans. It affects predominantly women (80 percent) and is usually realized after the onset of middle age. Osteoporosis is known as a "silent disease" because there are frequently no symptoms until a bone fracture occurs.

Essentially, osteoporosis is bone loss. Bones are living, growing tissues. They are made mostly of collagen, a protein that provides a soft framework, and calcium phosphate, a mineral that adds strength and hardens the framework. More than 99 percent of the body's calcium is contained in the bones and teeth.

An inadequate supply of calcium over a lifetime is thought to play a significant role in the development of osteoporosis as people age. Many published studies show that low calcium intake appears to be associated with low bone mass, rapid bone loss, and high fracture rates.

Calcium may be present in your diet, and you may even be taking calcium supplements; however, your bones may not be absorbing the calcium. It takes more than the presence of calcium in your body to have strong bones. The calcium has to be properly metabolized in order to become bone. Your body needs healthy levels of magnesium, vitamin B_6, vitamin D_3, and the mineral boron to build strong bones.

Xylitol's Role in Bone Building

A recent study done by researchers in Finland on rats with deficient bone mineral density showed that the dietary supplementation of calcium with the addition of Xylitol is more effective in increasing bone density than calcium alone. While more research needs to be carried out on Xylitol's ability to aid in calcium reabsorption and increased bone density, this is certainly a promising sign.

Linda Built Bone with Xylitol

About three years ago, I was only just beginning to use Xylitol in my practice. Many women came to see me because they had a diagnosis of osteopenia (early osteoporosis) or osteoporosis. I'd been quite successful in treating those conditions, usually recommending particular diets and calcium supplementation.

One particular patient, Linda, came to see me for help in treating her osteopenia. As I did for most of my other patients, I started her on a diet high in the green vegetables that contain calcium. She began taking all of the nutritional supplements that have been known to stop osteoporosis in its tracks, including natural hormone replacement therapy, and she was doing weight-bearing exercises on a regular basis. Linda was able to stop her bone loss but was unable to grow new bone. Then came Xylitol.

Linda went on "the Xylitol diet" to lose ten pounds. At the time, I had not seen studies that reported Xylitol promoted bone remineralization, so I never expected it to make a difference. But Linda loved the taste of Xylitol and felt better not eating sugar, so she kept it as a permanent part of her diet.

Six months later, Linda went for a bone density test. She came back to see me very excited. "My bone density test has finally improved," Linda said. "What could have finally done it?" At the time, I didn't know, but now I strongly suspect that Xylitol helped. Linda, if you are reading this book, keep eating Xylitol!

TOOTH DECAY

It may sound odd to be told that a sweetener can actually prevent tooth decay. After all, if you've ever had a cavity, one of the first things your dentist tells you is to stay away from the sweets. Xylitol, you will learn, is the exception to many rules. To understand how Xylitol improves dental health, however, it is important to first understand how tooth decay actually occurs.

Bacteria are normally present in the mouth. The bacteria convert all foods—especially sugar and starch—into acids. Bacteria, acid, food debris, and saliva combine in the mouth to form a sticky substance called plaque that adheres to the teeth. It is most prominent on the grooved chewing surfaces of back molars, just above the gum line on all teeth, and at the edges of fillings. Plaque that is not removed from the teeth mineralizes into tartar. Plaque and tartar irritate the gums, resulting in gingivitis and ultimately periodontitis.

The acids in plaque dissolve the enamel surface of the tooth and create holes in the tooth (cavities). Cavities are usually painless until they grow very large inside the internal structures of the tooth (the dentin and the pulp at the core) and can cause death of the nerve and blood vessels in the tooth. If left untreated, a tooth abscess can develop.

Plaque and bacteria begin to accumulate within twenty minutes after eating, the time when most bacterial activity occurs. If plaque and bacteria are left on the teeth, cavities can develop and untreated tooth decay can result in death of the internal structures of the tooth and ultimately the loss of the tooth.

Dietary sugars and starches (carbohydrates) increase the risk of tooth decay. The type of carbohydrate and the timing and frequency of ingestion are more important than the amount. Sticky foods are more harmful than nonsticky foods because they remain on the surface of the teeth. Frequent snacking increases the time that acids are in contact with the surface of the tooth.

Xylitol's Dental Connection

- Xylitol inhibits plaque and dental caries by 80 percent.

- Xylitol retards demineralization of tooth enamel.

- Xylitol promotes remineralization of tooth enamel by binding with calcium.

- Xylitol increases saliva production.

- Xylitol relieves dry mouth (a frequent problem for the elderly and those who use many prescription drugs).

- Xylitol has a protein-stabilizing effect to improve breath odor.

- Xylitol reduces infections in the mouth and periodontal (gum) disease by not allowing bacteria to adhere to *epithelial cells* (a thin protective layer of cells lining the mouth).

- *Streptococcus mutans* (strep bacteria) are the beginning of tooth decay. These bacteria live in the high-acid environment of the mouth. They adhere to teeth, eat through the enamel, and cause plaque to form and cause tooth decay. Xylitol is alkaline (the opposite of acid), making the mouth an unfriendly place for strep bacteria to live. Chewing Xylitol gum regularly creates a long-lasting change in the bacteria of the mouth.

I find that all the "Xylitol-prevents-tooth-decay" talk is 100-percent true. My dentist says so, and I personally know so. I have not had a cavity in the four years since I began chewing Xylitol-sweetened gum. And with the busy life I lead, it was a pleasure to give up carrying a toothbrush and toothpaste in order to brush after every meal. I no longer floss and use water picks in the ladies room, and I threw out that awful tasting mouthwash. (I don't suggest this for you unless you get your dentist's okay.)

I brush my teeth in the morning and before I go to bed (for two minutes—timed by my electric toothbrush). I also chew Xylitol gum or mints after each meal, before bed, and upon rising. I have the same or better results than I did with the toothpaste and floss in the ladies room. I know that my teeth and breath are clean because Xylitol kills bacteria in my mouth and prevents plaque from forming on my teeth.

MIDDLE EAR INFECTIONS IN CHILDREN

Middle ear infections (otitis media) occur when there is bacterial or viral infection of the fluid of the middle ear, which causes production of fluid or pus. On some occasions, bacteria can actually be spread from the mouth to the ear through the eustachian tube, which connects the oral cavity to the middle ear. Middle ear infections are more common in children because their eustachian tubes are shorter, narrower, and more horizontal than in adults.

Xylitol's Middle Ear Connection

As mentioned earlier, Xylitol gum and mints are great preventive therapy for knocking out infections that begin in the mouth. This is due to the alkaline environment that it creates in the mouth. Remember, strep bacteria cannot grow in an alkaline environment. Bacterial infections that could spread from the mouth to the ear no longer happen. Studies have found that if children chew Xylitol gum for five minutes after every meal, it will help prevent ear infections.

A study done in Oulu, Finland, involved 306 Finnish children. They were given gum sweetened with either sucrose (table sugar) or Xylitol. The average age of the children was five years old, and most had recurrent middle ear infections. At the end of two months, the group chewing Xylitol gum had a 40 percent decrease in the incidence of middle ear infections compared with those who chewed the sugar-sweetened gum. In other studies, children who chewed Xylitol-sweetened gum were compared with children who did not chew gum. The Xylitol gum chewers had fewer ear infections. Scientists now believe that other infections that begin in the mouth (sinus and lung infections) can be curtailed by chewing Xylitol gum and mints.

CANDIDA ALBICANS AND OTHER YEAST AND BACTERIA

Candida albicans is normally found in small amounts in the vagina, the mouth, the digestive tract, and on the skin without causing disease or symptoms. Candida is an opportunistic infection, and usually poses the biggest problems when the body's immunity is compromised in some way.

If you have ever had a yeast infection, such as Candida, you will remember that the first food removed from your diet was sugar. Sugar isn't just a breeding ground for bacteria in your mouth. When you swallow sugar, its high-acid environment moves to your gut. Here, unhealthy bacteria are bred and colonize, and then travel throughout your body. Have you ever felt gassy or bloated after eating a meal high in sugar and other refined carbohydrates? I'm sure most of you can relate.

Xylitol's Role as a Yeast Killer

More than 70 percent of the patients who come to see me for the first time have problems with intestinal yeast (mostly from eating diets high in simple sugars). In the past, I had to remove sweets from their diets. Now sweets (in the form of Xylitol) are part of their prescription for health. This is only one small way in which Xylitol has helped my patients become healthier.

Jonathan Wright, M.D., a well-known practitioner of integrative medicine, suggests that we use Xylitol as a preventive measure. He says that disease begins with bacteria, and although drug companies develop antibiotics to kill bacteria, all of them are not killed. He points out that as fast as the drug companies develop antibiotics, bacteria develop new ways to outsmart the drugs. Dr. Wright suggests that it is better to destroy the bacteria before they have a chance to attach to the body. Eating Xylitol is one way to do this.

XYLITOL AND SPORTS NUTRITION

Strength athletes searching for alternatives to steroids are particularly intrigued by Xylitol. Even thin runners want to avoid the "emaciated" look caused by upper body protein being used for fuel. Developing lean muscle mass involves increasing anabolism (muscle building) while minimizing catabolism (muscle breakdown). There are well-documented Xylitol effects in conditions of stress and trauma. It is not yet known how well these findings will translate for athletes and bodybuilders, but the possibilities look promising.

According to Dr. John Peldyak, a dentist who is at the forefront of Xylitol research, there are a number of characteristics of Xylitol that make it an appealing choice for strength athletes. Its low glycemic index and mostly insulin-independent metabolism make it ideal for maintaining steady blood sugar and insulin levels. This may help promote muscle building. Through its use with severely traumatized patients, Xylitol has been shown to have a muscle-sparing effect (anticatabolism). It is also a precursor to key antioxidants, which minimize free-radical damage generated by severe exercise. Because Xylitol is efficiently and steadily converted to glucose (sugar used immediately for energy) and glycogen (stored carbohydrates for later use), it may be particularly useful when coupled with other carbohydrates for recovery after heavy exercise. Likewise, it may be valuable for carbohydrate-loading (supercompensating) by packing glycogen after a depletion phase.

XYLITOL AS AN ANTIOXIDANT

The health-promoting properties of Xylitol as an antioxidant have only just begun to be explored. As mentioned previously, Xylitol is a precursor to antioxidants. Dr. Peldyak states, "An important added bonus of *Xylitol* metabolism is the activation of the glutathione antioxidant system, which helps to squelch free radicals generated by heavy exercise, thereby reducing oxidative damage to muscle and blood cells." Continued studies into Xylitol's role as an antioxidant are certainly warranted.

BREAKING THE SUGAR ADDICTION WITH XYLITOL

We are unaccustomed to thinking of sweet foods as healthy foods. I often notice the resistance and disbelief of my patients when I ask them to go on "The Sweet Miracle of Xylitol Diet" (see Chapter 3). But it is not long before they call to thank me, saying things like, "I thought this was a crazy idea. I figured eating sweets would touch off my sugar cravings, but it hasn't happened. Now I don't want to eat sugar. Why?"

I answer them by explaining that in many cases, sugar is an addictive food. As with other addictive substances, eating sugar causes you to want more. The sweet taste of it is nice, but the insulin reaction it sets off in your body is the physiological basis for addiction.

When your blood sugar level rises, you feel energized and happy (even euphoric). When the level drops, you can feel depressed, exhausted, and hungry for sugary foods. You eat them, crave more, and it becomes a vicious cycle.

If we eat sweet foods made from Xylitol, we eliminate the blood sugar reaction because Xylitol does not cause our blood sugar to rise. Sweet food becomes "just another food" without an addictive body-wide response.

XYLITOL, THE GLYCEMIC INDEX, AND THE LOSS OF BODY FAT

The Glycemic Index Diet is a popular book that was published in Australia. The glycemic index is a ranking of foods on a scale of 0 to 100, based upon the amount they cause blood sugar to rise during digestion, with glucose ranking 100. The theory behind it is that high-fiber foods digest more slowly than low-fiber foods. Simple carbohydrates like sugar are lower in fiber, so they digest quickly. The longer it takes food to be digested, the less impact the food has on insulin and the healthier the food is. Simple carbohydrates like sugar digest quickly in the mouth and set off an instant insulin reaction in the body. Dr. Paul Zimmet of the International Diabetes Institute in Melbourne, Australia, describes the glycemic index (GI) as "an established physiologically based method to classify foods according to their glucose-raising potential. It compares the level of *glycemia* (sugar level in blood) after equal carbohydrate portion foods and ranks them relative to a standard (usually glucose or white bread). When ranked against sugar, which is 100, Xylitol measures 7— a dramatic difference."

As a result of this low GI number, when you eat Xyiltol, your body does not secrete insulin. When insulin is not available to the body, the body begins to burn body fat. When you eat carbohydrates (like sugar and starch), your insulin levels rise, forcing your body to use dietary carbohydrates instead of stored body fat for energy. Not only does Xylitol not cause an insulin reaction in your body, it is a natural insulin stabilizer.

A recent study examined the metabolic response of Xylitol in eight healthy, nonobese men, after an overnight fast. In this study, the researchers examined the glucose (blood sugar), insulin, and C-peptide responses and changes in carbohydrate and lipid oxidation after the ingestion of 25 grams of either lactitol, Xylitol, or glucose. After the ingestion of lactitol or Xylitol, the rise in glucose, insulin, and C-peptide concentrations was less than after the ingestion of glucose, with no difference between lactitol and Xylitol. Reactive hypoglycemia was observed three hours after glucose ingestion, but not after the ingestion of the two sugar alcohols.

In an earlier study, Xylitol, taken by mouth in solution as a single 30-gram dose, produced only a minimal rise in blood glucose and no rise in plasma insulin concentration. Glucose in similar doses, on the other hand,

3.

The Sweet Miracle
of Xylitol Diet

How good would an alternative sweetener be if you could not lose or at least control your weight while enjoying it? Not so good. Xylitol is better than good—it's a "sweet miracle."

When I first began using Xylitol in my practice, I decided to put some of my patients (those who had been having the most difficulty giving up sugar) on a diet that included a generous amount of Xylitol sweets. Ten patients began and finished the three-week diet. They used the recipes that begin on page 56 to make and enjoy decadently delicious Xylitol-sweetened desserts.

In addition, the dieters chewed Xylitol gum or mints between meals. This advice came from Dr. Peldyak's book, *Xylitol: Sweeten Your Smile.* He wrote, "Xylitol is useful between meal treats to maintain a steady trickle of energy. Unabsorbed Xylitol acts like dietary fiber, helping to maintain healthy gut function. Partial bacterial fermentation here produces volatile short chain fatty acids, which are utilized along existing insulin-independent energy pathways."

Each week, when patients came in to be weighed,

they were given new recipes for the following week. I also reminded them to buy Xylitol-sweetened mints and gum to use between meals. Let their stories help you decide on a course of action.

PATIENT OUTCOMES

Bill and Sally's Experience

Bill is a cancer survivor who presently has diabetes and hypertension. When he agreed to go on the Xylitol diet, he had been uncontrollably binging on sweets. He was overweight, had a high fasting glucose (about 190), and elevated blood pressure (200/150). His doctor had urged him to either go on a diet or begin to take stronger drugs to control his glucose and blood pressure levels.

Meanwhile, Bill's wife, Sally, had been struggling to lose five pounds. She felt that she could support Bill by going on the Xylitol diet with him. They began the diet together. Sally reported having to watch Bill carefully at the beginning. "He would sneak sugar from a sugar bowl in a restaurant!" she reported.

At the end of the first week, Sally had lost one pound and Bill had gained two pounds. Sally reported having more energy, which she claimed she needed to keep a check on Bill's sugar cheating. By the second week's end, Sally reported that Bill was now eating Xylitol from the sugar bowl. He had lost the two pounds he had gained, plus one-half pound more. Sally had lost two pounds. At the end of the third week, Bill was completely off sugar and reported that his sugar cravings were gone. His blood pressure had dropped to 150/90, and he had lost five pounds in total. Sally had lost one more pound, leaving her one pound from her goal.

Olga's Experience

Olga had been my patient for at least a year and had not lost weight. She loved sugar. I wondered why she kept coming back. I felt that she must still have hopes of losing the thirty-five pounds that she originally came to lose. I offered her the Xylitol diet. She was excited about it because it meant that she could eat sweet foods.

Olga surprised me. By the end of the first week, she had lost five pounds. I asked her what she had done. "I only ate dessert," Olga replied. "It was great!" I didn't think it was so great, but she loved it. She promised me that she would introduce salads to her diet in the coming week.

The second week passed and Olga came back an additional one and a half pounds lighter. She had only eaten two salads that week! I had created a dessert monster!

I was relieved when she came in to be weighed at the end of the third week. Olga had lost two more pounds. "My sweet cravings are gone. I hardly baked this week at all. I was able to follow the diet, chewing the gum and eating the mints. I only baked one dessert that I ate three times," she declared.

Olga went on to lose all of her weight. The last time I saw her, she had kept it off for two years.

Tony's Experience

Although Tony gained five pounds on the Xylitol diet, his

is still a success story. He was not overweight, but came to me because he was a tired bodybuilder. At thirty, he felt like he was rapidly aging. He would load up on carbohydrates all day so that he would have enough energy to work out. I told him about the diet, and he asked to go on it. I had no idea what would happen, but I knew that it would not hurt him.

After his first three days on the diet, he reported that he felt miserable—even more tired and weak. On the third day, he couldn't even get out of bed. I felt that he was experiencing serious sugar withdrawal and gave him the choice of going off the diet.

However, he chose to stay with it, and by day five, he was feeling great. He began lifting weights again. I suggested that he eat a larger amount of protein and vegetables than the others on the diet.

By the end of the first week, Tony had lost two pounds. He reported having more energy to train for short periods. By the end of the second week, he said that he felt great and was going skydiving. At the end of a month, Tony weighed five pounds more than when he began the diet, but it was all muscle. "Look at my arm muscle," he said as he flexed. "Thank you so much for helping me 'kick the sugar habit.'"

Mimi's Experience

Mimi was a spunky eighty-two-year-old woman. Her beau had asked her to be his date at his granddaughter's wedding, and she wanted to look her best. She confided, "I want to knock 'em dead!"

The first week, she did not completely understand the Xylitol diet, and ate a few things that were not on it, like fruit and her morning oatmeal. She weighed the same and was obviously disappointed. After we discussed her slips, she understood the diet completely. The next week, she strictly adhered to the diet but lost only one-half pound. I commented that she looked less round than the one-half pound would indicate. We decided to take her measurements to be able to compare them in the future.

After this second visit, Mimi went to visit her son in New York for a month. When she returned, she looked wonderful. "My beau said that I was the prettiest eighty-two year old in the Hamptons," Mimi reported. I noticed that she had a diamond ring on her engagement finger. "We are engaged," she said. "He can't take his hands off of me."

Although Mimi had only lost three pounds, her measurements revealed that she had lost four inches around her waist.

Mimi also enjoyed another benefit of Xylitol. She had been having a troublesome time with her gums. They had been bleeding and blistering. "My gums are better," Mimi reported. "My dentist said that my gums are pink and healthy. She wanted to know what I had done. I told her about Xylitol."

Harriet and John's Experience

The stories of Harriet and John were uneventful, but their results weren't. Harriet lost four pounds and John lost five pounds while they were on the Xylitol diet!

Martha and June's Experience

Martha and June were a mother and daughter who had been competing to lose weight for months. The daughter, June, was ahead by seven pounds but was getting bored with her diet. I thought that adding sweets would make it more interesting. Martha decided to change her diet, too, because she wasn't getting the desired results from the diet she was on. They both agreed to go on the Xylitol diet.

By the third week, Martha had lost five pounds, but June's weight had stayed the same. I am not quite sure why. June may have been overeating the Xylitol sweets. Remember, anything in excess is unhealthy—even too many Xylitol-sweetened treats. On the other hand, Martha didn't like to bake so she wasn't eating any of the "goodies." She followed the prescribed diet, but her only treats were the mints and gum.

Martha experienced another interesting result. Even after the diet, she continued to eat the gum and mints because she liked them so much. Six months later, she called to tell me that her bone density had improved. She wondered if the Xylitol could have facilitated the strengthening of her bones. "There are studies supporting that," I replied.

Zelda's Experience

Zelda could not give up sugar long enough to allow the Xylitol to end her sugar cravings. She came in once to be weighed (at the end of the three weeks) only because I pestered her until she did. She had added the Xylitol to her regular diet and had gained two pounds. Zelda's experience reinforces the fact that Xylitol can't perform its "sweet miracle" if sugar is not eliminated from the diet.

In Sweet Summation

This ten-person study reinforced my belief that insulin resistance is a major part of weight gain. When sugar and most of the other carbohydrates are removed from your diet, your body can behave normally, and you will be able to lose excess weight. Nine of the patients in the study did exceptionally well. Of course, this was a short-term clinical study and none of the subjects were grossly overweight.

Perhaps you are thinking that you could do exceptionally well on the Xylitol diet. Try it out for three weeks and see how you do. Simply follow the suggestions on the following pages.

THE THREE-WEEK "SWEET MIRACLE" DIET

WEEK ONE

- Drink 8 glasses of spring water each day.

- Take 4 multivitamins (any brand) each day.

- Take 4 flaxseed oil soft gels (or $1\frac{1}{2}$ tablespoons of ground flaxseeds) each day.

Breakfast

- 2 eggs prepared as you like, or an egg-white omelet made with your choice of cheeses, vegetables, or meats.

- 1 Morning Sunflower Biscuit (page 62) with coffee, tea, or another warm beverage.

- Every hour between breakfast and lunch, chew two pieces of Xylitol gum or eat two Xylitol mints.**

Lunch

- A large green salad with chicken, fish, or meat and sugar-free or Xylitol-sweetened dressing.

- 1 serving Xylitol-sweetened ice cream (pages 56–58) and a sugar-free beverage of your choice.

- Every hour between lunch and dinner, chew two pieces of Xylitol-sweetened gum or eat two Xylitol mints.**

Dinner

- A high-protein entrée such as lamb or beef.

- 1 cup of a green vegetable steamed or sautéed in butter, extra virgin olive oil, or coconut oil, seasoned to your taste.

- 2 Xylitol-sweetened cookies (pages 59–66) and a sugar-free hot beverage of your choice.

- Before bed, chew 2 pieces of Xylitol-sweetened gum or eat 4 Xylitol mints.**

**If you are a first-time Xylitol user and you go on the "Xylitol binge," you can expect a "cleansing" result. Earlier you learned that eating large amounts of Xylitol can cause diarrhea until the Xylitol-digesting enzymes in your body become accustomed to your intake. The "enzyme awakening" could take up to ten days. You can think of the diarrhea as a way to cleanse your digestive tract, or you can begin eating Xylitol more slowly (two desserts spread over a day).

WEEK TWO

- Drink 8 glasses of spring water each day.

- Take 4 multivitamins (any brand) each day.

- Take 4 flaxseed oil soft gels (or $1\frac{1}{2}$ tablespoons of ground flaxseeds) each day.

Breakfast

- 2 ounces of cheese and 1 Wasa Rye Crisp Bread or $\frac{1}{2}$ cup oatmeal with one tablespoon butter.

- $\frac{1}{4}$ cup Coffee Sorbet (page 58) or coffee with cream and Xylitol.

- Every hour between breakfast and lunch, chew 2 pieces of Xylitol gum or eat 2 Xylitol mints.

Lunch

- 1 cup tuna, egg, salmon, or chicken salad (with mayo or olive oil) on a bed of greens.

- 2 Xylitol-sweetened cookies (pages 59–66) and a beverage of your choice.

- Every hour between lunch and dinner, chew 2 pieces of Xylitol gum or eat 4 Xylitol mints.

Dinner

- As many protein servings and green vegetables as you wish.

- 1 slice Xylitol-sweetened dessert of your choice.

- Before bed, eat 4 Xylitol mints.

——— WEEK THREE ———

- Drink 8 glasses of spring water each day.

- Take 4 multivitamins (any brand) each day.

- Take 4 flaxseed oil soft gels (or 1½ tablespoons of ground flaxseeds) each day.

- Every hour between breakfast and lunch, chew 2 pieces of Xylitol gum or eat 2 Xylitol mints.

- Every hour between lunch and dinner, chew 2 pieces of Xylitol gum or eat 2 Xylitol mints.

- Before bed, eat 4 Xylitol mints.

- Choose foods freely from the following list and eat them in any order you wish. You don't have to eat everything listed.

FOOD LIST FOR WEEK THREE

1–2 cups of green vegetables per day

2 eggs per day

1 ounce of butter per day

2 ounces of cheese per day

3 cups of salad greens per day

4 tablespoons of olive or coconut oil per day

2 tablespoons of vinegar per day

Juice of 2 lemons per day

2 tablespoons of heavy cream or half-and-half per day

2 ounces of soymilk per day

½ cup oatmeal per day

2 Wasa Crisp Breads per day

A variety of meat, poultry, or fish per day

Any 3 Xylitol sweets per day

4 teaspoons of Xylitol per day

½ cup berries per day

RECIPES FOR THE "SWEET MIRACLE" DIET

The following recipes contain carbohydrates in the form of unbleached flour. Please be careful not to eat more of them than you are allowed on the diet. Although your body will not have an insulin reaction to the Xylitol, flour will cause your body to produce insulin. Protein powder, which won't increase blood glucose levels, can be used in place of flour if you are an inventive cook. You can also choose soy and spelt, which have less of an effect on blood glucose levels, or flaxseed flour, which may be difficult to come by. None of these can be substituted cup-for-cup for white flour. If you are insulin resistant, choose the recipes with the least amount of flour. You will not feel cheated; all of the recipes are delicious.

Frozen Desserts

GINGER ICE CREAM

MAKES 5 $\frac{1}{2}$-CUP SERVINGS.

For easy preparation you will need:

- Small saucepan • Wire whisk
- Ice-cream maker

Ginger Mixture

2 inches of fresh ginger root,
peeled and thinly sliced

1 cup water

Ice Cream

$\frac{1}{2}$ cup ground ginger mixture

2 cups heavy cream

$\frac{1}{4}$ cup Xylitol

1. To make the ginger mixture, combine ginger root and water in a saucepan. Bring to a boil and reduce heat to a simmer. Allow to simmer until the liquid reduces to $\frac{1}{2}$ cup. Cool. Place in a food processor and grind.

2. Mix together the ginger mixture, heavy cream, and Xylitol. Place in an ice-cream maker and churn to freeze. (The ice-cream maker will stop when the ice cream is frozen.)

GINGER ICE MILK

MAKES 10 ¹/₄-CUP SERVINGS.

For easy preparation you will need:

- Small saucepan
- Wire whisk
- Ice-cream maker

Ginger Mixture

2 inches of fresh ginger root,
peeled and thinly sliced

1 cup water

Ice Milk

¹/₂ cup ground ginger mixture

2 cups unsweetened rice milk or soymilk

¹/₄ cup Xylitol (or more to taste)

1. To make the ginger mixture, combine ginger root and water in a saucepan. Bring to a boil and reduce heat to a simmer. Allow to simmer until the liquid reduces to ¹/₂ cup. Cool. Place in a food processor and grind.

2. Mix together the ginger mixture, milk, and Xylitol. Place in an ice-cream maker and churn to freeze. (The ice-cream maker will stop when the ice milk is frozen.)

COFFEE ICE CREAM

MAKES 5 $1/2$-CUP SERVINGS.

> *For easy preparation you will need:*
> - Small saucepan   • Wire whisk
>   - Ice-cream maker

2 tablespoons instant coffee crystals
$1/2$ cup half-and-half
6 tablespoons Xylitol
1 teaspoon coffee extract
2 cups heavy cream

1. Warm coffee crystals and half-and-half in saucepan until coffee crystals melt. Whisk in Xylitol and coffee extract. Allow to cool in refrigerator for fifteen minutes.

2. Whisk coffee mixture into heavy cream. Place in ice-cream maker and churn to freeze. (The ice-cream maker will stop when the ice cream is frozen.)

Variation:

For Coffee Sorbet, which is lower in calories (but higher in carbohydrates), follow the Coffee Ice Cream recipe but substitute 2 cups of skimmed milk for the heavy cream.

Cookies, Bars, & Biscuits

——— LEMON SHORTBREAD BARS ———

MAKES **27** 1-INCH-X-**3**-INCH BARS.

For easy preparation you will need:
- Electric mixer with bowl
- Measuring spoons
- 9-inch square nonstick baking pan, buttered
- Wire cooling rack

6 ounces of sweet butter

2 teaspoons lemon rind, grated

$3/4$ cup Xylitol, rubbed through a fine strainer

2 cups unbleached flour

1 tablespoon lemon juice

1. Preheat the oven to 325°F.

2. Place butter, lemon rind, and all but 2 tablespoons of Xylitol in bowl. Beat until butter is light and fluffy. Add flour and lemon juice. Blend well. Roll mixture into a firm ball and press into buttered baking pan.

3. Bake at 325°F for thirty-five minutes or until browned. Cut into 1-inch by 3-inch bars and place on a rack to cool. Serve bars dusted with remaining 2 tablespoons of Xylitol.

── NUTTY, FRUITY OAT COOKIES ──

MAKES 16 COOKIES.

For easy preparation you will need:

- Medium-sized saucepan
- Wooden spoon
- Handheld electric mixer
- 2 nonstick cookie sheets
- Wire cooling rack
- Measuring spoons

2 ounces of sweet butter

$1/4$ cup creamy peanut butter

$1/2$ cup unbleached flour

1 teaspoon baking powder

$1/2$ cup rolled oats

$1/4$ cup dried apricots, chopped

$3/4$ cup unsalted roasted peanuts

$1/2$ cup Xylitol

1 small egg, lightly beaten

1. Preheat the oven to 350°F.

2. Combine butter and peanut butter in saucepan. Stir over low heat until butter is melted. Remove from heat. Using the hand mixer on low speed, beat in remaining ingredients until a smooth batter forms. Drop by tablespoonfuls onto cookie sheet, about two inches apart.

3. Bake at 350°F for twelve minutes or until browned. Remove to cooling rack. Cool on cookie sheets.

MACADAMIA COOKIES

MAKES ABOUT 16 COOKIES.

For easy preparation you will need:

- Electric mixer fitted with small bowl
- 2 nonstick cookie sheets, buttered
- Measuring spoons
- Wire cooling rack

1 ounce sweet butter, melted

1 tablespoon honey

$1/4$ cup Xylitol

$1/2$ teaspoon baking soda

$1/2$ cup unsweetened, shredded coconut
(available in health-food stores)

$3/4$ cups unbleached flour

3 tablespoons macadamia nuts,
finely chopped

1. Preheat the oven to 350°F.

2. Combine butter, honey, Xylitol, and baking soda in small bowl. Beat until smooth. Add coconut, flour, and macadamias. Beat on a low speed until well blended. Roll rounded teaspoons of mixture into balls, and place on cookie sheets (about two inches apart). Press center of each cookie with floured fork.

3. Bake at 350°F for ten minutes or until browned. Allow cookies to remain in oven for five minutes after turning off oven before removing to cooling rack.

— Morning Sunflower Biscuits —

MAKES 15 BISCUITS.

For easy preparation you will need:

- Electric mixer fitted with small bowl   • Measuring spoons
- 2 nonstick cookie sheets, buttered

2 ounces of sweet butter
at room temperature

1 teaspoon lemon rind, grated

1 teaspoon orange rind, grated

½ cup Xylitol

1 small egg

¾ cup unbleached flour

¼ cup unsweetened shredded coconut
(available in health-food stores)

¼ cup sunflower seeds, toasted

1. Preheat the oven to 350°F.

2. Beat butter, rinds, Xylitol, and egg in small bowl until smooth. Stir in the flour, coconut, and sunflower seeds.

3. Drop by tablespoonfuls onto cookie sheet, about two inches apart. Flatten slightly with a floured fork.

4. Bake at 350°F for twenty minutes or until browned. Remove from oven and allow to completely cool on rack before removing the biscuits from cookie sheet.

COCONUT TULLES
(THIN COCONUT "SHELL" COOKIES)

MAKES 12 COOKIES.

For easy preparation you will need:

- Electric mixer fitted with small bowl
- Teaspoon
- 2 nonstick cookie sheets, lightly buttered
- Flat spatula
- Rolling pin

1 egg white

¼ cup Xylitol

2 tablespoons unbleached flour

2 tablespoons sweet butter at room temperature

¼ teaspoon coconut extract

2 tablespoons unsweetened shredded coconut

1. Preheat the oven to 350°F.

2. Beat egg white in a small bowl until soft peaks form. Gradually add Xylitol, beating the mixture between additions to dissolve the sweetener. Add flour, butter, and coconut extract. Beat until smooth.

3. Drop one level tablespoon of mixture onto buttered cookie sheet. Spread mixture into a circle. Leaving about two inches between cookies, continue until all the batter is used. Sprinkle each cookie with shredded coconut.

4. Bake at 350°F for five to eight minutes (or until cookies are lightly browned). Remove from oven. Slide a spatula under cookie, lift off cookie sheet, and quickly shape over a rolling pin until firm.

── CHINESE ALMOND COOKIES ──

MAKES 14 COOKIES.

For easy preparation you will need:

- Electric mixer fitted with small bowl
- 2 nonstick cookie sheets, buttered
- Measuring spoons   • Wire cooling rack

---

4 ounces of sweet butter, chopped

$1/2$ cup Xylitol

1 cup unbleached flour

2 teaspoons baking powder

$1/4$ cup ground almonds

4 tablespoons sliced almonds

1. Preheat the oven to 400°F.

2. Beat butter and Xylitol in bowl of electric mixer until smooth. Stir in flour, baking powder, and ground nuts. Roll level teaspoons of mixture into balls and place on buttered cookie sheet (leaving about two inches between cookies). Flatten slightly with a floured fork. Place sliced almonds on top of cookies.

3. Bake at 400°F for ten minutes or until browned. Remove from oven to cooling rack. Allow to cool five minutes before removing from cookie sheets.

— CHOCOLATE-PISTACHIO BISCOTTI —

MAKES 24 BISCOTTI.

For easy preparation you will need:

- Electric mixer fitted with small bowl
- 2 nonstick cookie sheets, buttered
- Floured board for kneading
- Wire cooling rack
- Measuring spoons • Sharp serrated knife
- Loaf pan lined with parchment paper, buttered

$3/4$ cup Xylitol

1 egg

$3/4$ cup unbleached flour

$1/2$ teaspoon baking powder

$1/2$ cup shelled pistachios, toasted

$1/4$ cup unsweetened cocoa

1 tablespoon Xylitol

1. Preheat the oven to 350°F.

2. Using low speed, mix Xylitol and egg together in small bowl. Add flour, baking powder, and pistachios. Mix until soft dough forms. Remove from mixer.

3. Divide dough into two portions. Knead first portion on lightly floured board until smooth but still slightly sticky. Divide this portion into two more pieces. Roll each of the two pieces into a log shape (long enough to fit the length of the loaf pan). Set aside.

4. Mix cocoa and one tablespoon of Xylitol together. Knead the cocoa mixture into the remaining dough until smooth. Divide into two pieces. Roll each of the pieces into a log shape (long enough to fit the length of the loaf pan). Gently press the logs together (one without cocoa and one with the cocoa) side by side in the loaf pan.

5. Bake at 350°F for thirty-five minutes or until dry. Remove loaf pan from oven to cooling rack. Cool logs for ten minutes on rack.

6. Turn oven down to 275°F. Using a serrated knife, slice each log diagonally to make twelve slices. Place slices flat on cookie sheets and bake at 275°F for thirty minutes until slices are dry. Cool ten minutes on cooling rack before removing biscotti.

4.

Frequently Asked Questions about Xylitol

Most consumers in the United States have never heard of Xylitol or have only a very vague idea of what it is and what it can do. The following pages summarize the key attributes of this little-known product. For those of you who have read through this book thoroughly, this will serve mainly as a review, but it may also answer a few lingering questions you may have about this "sweet miracle."

Q. Why has Xylitol, a food additive fully approved by the FDA, been kept a secret all of these years?

A. If you live in the United States, Xylitol may seem like a secret to you. However it has been used commercially in Europe and Asia for more than forty years. Until recently, it has been more costly than sugar, so we have not embraced its use in this country. Fortunately, the prices have recently come down.

Q. **Is it true that Xylitol is all natural?**

A. Yes. Our own bodies produce it during normal glucose metabolism. It also occurs naturally in berries, some vegetables, and woody substances, such as birch bark and corncobs.

Q. **Where does the Xylitol I buy in the store come from?**

A. The Xylitol that you buy in stores is most probably processed from either birch bark or corncobs.

Q. **I have heard that Xylitol looks and tastes teaspoon-for-teaspoon like sugar. Is that true?**

A. Yes, Xylitol is produced in a crystallized form (like sugar) and can be substituted for sugar in recipes teaspoon-for-teaspoon.

Q. **Can I add Xylitol to hot and cold beverages and expect it to sweeten them like sugar does?**

A. Yes, Xylitol will sweeten anything you eat or drink exactly the way sugar does.

Q. **Most sugar alternatives have an aftertaste. What is Xylitol's aftertaste?**

A. During and after eating Xylitol, the taste in your mouth is exactly like table sugar.

Q. Is Xylitol as likely to cause me to gain weight as sugar is?

A. Xylitol has 40 percent fewer calories and 75 percent fewer carbohydrates than sugar—making it a nutritive, reduced-calorie, and low-carbohydrate sugar alternative. And it offers weight-loss benefits (because it helps to stabilize insulin) that sugar and most other sugar alternatives do not offer.

Q. How does Xylitol help with weight loss?

A. Xylitol ranks a 7 on the glycemic index (table sugar is 100). The glycemic index measures the ability of a food to raise insulin levels. Since Xylitol does not raise insulin levels, you can eat sweet foods containing Xylitol without experiencing blood sugar fluctuations. When your insulin is stable, you are much less likely to crave sweet foods. Eating Xylitol allows sweet foods to become the same as any other foods you eat. It puts an end to sugar cravings and addiction. With the sugar addiction gone, you are once again in control of your eating. In addition, studies show that Xylitol may improve nitrogen balance in the body, and thereby help the body to burn fat.

Q. Does Xylitol have other health benefits?

A. Yes. The following are some of the health benefits we know about today, but scientists predict they will discover many more:

- It is a great way for people with diabetes to enjoy sweet foods since it is processed through the gut without involving insulin.

- It prevents tooth decay by inhibiting plaque and cavities by 80 percent.

- It promotes healthy bones by helping to remineralize bones.

- It makes the mouth and gut unfriendly environments for bacteria to live in.

Q. **Where can I buy Xylitol?**

A. You should be able to find Xylitol at your local health food store, but if you cannot, you can buy it on the World Wide Web. See the Appendix at the back of this book.

Conclusion

Knowledge is power. In these pages, you've gained invaluable knowledge about a natural product that most people have never even heard of, and now you have the power to use this knowledge to improve your health.

It seems that every time we open up a magazine or turn on the news, we hear of a new research study that states that an ever-increasing number of Americans (as much as 50 percent!) are obese. By now, we must realize that the standard high-carbohydrate, high-sugar American diet is just not healthy.

While using Xylitol may not be the only step you should take to break the unhealthy routine that many of us have become accustomed to, it certainly is an important one and is a great starting point. Remember, not only does using Xylitol spare you from the perilous consequences of eating sugar, but it actually makes you healthier. From helping you to lose weight to preventing diabetes to promoting dental health, Xylitol's benefits are undeniable. And if recent findings are any indication, all of its benefits have yet to be discovered.

I hope I've convinced you that adding Xylitol to your diet is a necessary, health-enhancing sweet experience. I consider it a miracle. It allows me the freedom to eat the sweet foods that I love and grow healthier. Having said that, all of the research, all of the case studies, and all of my high praises aren't nearly as persuasive as Xylitol itself. My best advice to you is to try it for a month or two and see if you notice any changes in your body and your health. I have no doubt that you will. I also have no doubt that once you see the power of Xylitol firsthand, it will become your sweetener of choice for life.

Appendix

Xylitol Products

As this "sweet miracle" becomes more popular, more companies will begin to offer Xylitol products. Meanwhile, here are some good sources you might want to check out. Be sure to ask about Xylitol at your local health food store, too.

Internet Sources for Xylitol

www.locarbdiner.com

www.perfectsweet.com

www.synergydiet.com

www.thesweetlifesweets.com

www.xylitolproducts.com

www.xylitolworks.com

Other Sources

Cledent Gum and Mints by Emerson Ecologics: 1-800-654-4432

Miracle Sweet/Allergy Research Group: 1-800-782-4274

References

Brunzell, JD. "Use of fructose, xylitol, or sorbitol as a sweetener in diabetes mellitus." *Diabetes Care* 1(1978):223–230.

Conclusion and review of the Michigan Xylitol Program 1986–1995 for the prevention of dental caries, 1996 FDI / World Dental Press.

Hauschildt, S, RA Chalmers, AM Lawson, K Schultis, and RW Watts. "Metabolic investigations after xylitol infusion in human subjects." *American Journal of Clinical Nutrition* 29(1976): 258–273.

Knuuttila, M. and Svancerg, M. "Preventative Effect of Xyltiol on Bone Ca in Ovariectomized Rats." *Connective Tissue Research* 28: 176.

Knuuttila, ML, et al. "Effects of dietary xylitol on collagen content and glycosylation in healthy and diabetic rats." *Life Sci.* 2000 Jun 8; 67(3): 283–90. PMID: 10983872 (PubMed—indexed for MedLine)

Kontiokari, Uhari, Koskela. "Antiadhesive effects of xylitol on otopathogenic bacteria." *Journal of Antimicrobial Chemotherapy* 41(1998): 563–565.

Life Sciences Research Office, 1986. Health aspects of sugar alcohols and lactose. Report prepared for the Center for Food Safety and Applied Nutrition, Food and Drug Administration, Washington, D.C., under contract No. FDA 223-83-2020 by the Life Sciences Research Office, Federation of American Societies for Experimental Biology (FASEB), Bethesda, MD.

Makinen, KK. "Dietary prevention of dental caries by xylitol—clinical effectiveness and safety." *Journal of Applied Nutrition* 44(1992): 16–28.

Makinen, KK, Soderling E. "Solubility of calcium salts, enamel, and hydroxyapatite in aqueous solutions of simple carbohydrates." *Calcified Tissue International* 36(1984): 64–71.

Mattila, PT, Svanberg MJ, Jamsa T, Knuuttila ML. "Improved bone biomechanical properties in xylitol-fed aged rats." *Metabolism* 51(1)(2002): 92–6.

Mattila, PT, Svanberg MJ, JKnuuttila ML. "Increased bone volume and bone mineral content in xylitol-fed aged rats." *Gerontology* 47(6)(2001): 300–5.

Mitchell, Allen A. "Xylitol Prophylaxis for Acute Otitis Media: *Tout de Suite?" Pediatrics* 102(1998): 974–975.

Natah, SS, KR Hussien, JA Tuominen, and VA Koivisto. "Metabolic response to lactitol and xylitol in healthy men." *American Journal of Clinical Nutrition* 65(1997): 947–950.

Office of the Federal Register, General Services Administration, 1987. Code of Federal Regulations. Title 21. S. 172. (395. Washington, D.C., U.S. Government Printing Office.

Olefsky, JM and P Crapo. "Fructose, xylitol, and sorbitol." *Diabetes Care* 3 (1980): 390–393.

Osteoporosis and Related Bone Diseases. *Promising Research Opportunities, National Coalition for Osteoporosis and Related Bone Disease.* Hogan & Hartson, Washington, DC.

Pauli, T, M Mattila, J Svanberg, P Pökkä, et al. "Dietary Xylitol Protects Against Weakening of Bone Biomechanical Properties in Ovariectomized Rats." *Journal of Nutrition.* 128(1998): 1811–1814.

Peldyak, John. *Xylitol, Sweeten Your Smile.* Mt. Pleasant, MI: Advanced Developments Inc., 1996.

Salminen, EK, SJ Salminen, L Porkka, P Kwasowski, V Marks, and PE Koivistoinen. "Xylitol vs glucose: effect on the rate of gastric emptying and motilin, insulin, and gastric inhibitory polypeptide release." *American Journal of Clinical Nutrition* 49(1989):1228–1232.

Scheinin, Arje, Kauko K., Makinen, Erkki Tammisalo, Maarit Rekola. "Turku sugar studies XVIII" *ACTA Odontologica Scandinavia* 33(1975): 269–278.

Shafer, RB, AS Levine, JM Marlette, and JE Morley. "Effects of xylitol on gastric emptying and food intake." *American Journal of Clinical Nutrition* 45(1987): 744–747.

Soderling, E, et al. "Effect of sorbitol, xylitol and xylitol/sorbitol chewing gums on dental plaque." *Carrier Res.* 1989; 23(5): 378–84. PMID: 2766327 (PubMed-indexed for MedLine).

Soderling, E, P Isokangas, K Pienihakkinen, and J Tenovuo. "Influence of Maternal Xylitol consumption on Acquisition of Mutans Steptococci by infants" *Journal of Dental Research* 79(3)(2000): 882–887.

Svanberg, M, M Knuuttila. Dietary xylitol prevents ovarectomy induced changes of bone in organic fractions in rats. *Bone and Mineral* 26(1994): 81–88.

Talbot, JM and KD Fisher. "The need for special foods and sugar substitutes by individuals with diabetes mellitus." *Diabetes Care* 1(1978): 231–240.

Terhi Tapiainen, Leevi Luotonen, Tero Kontiokari, Marjo Renko, and Matti Uhari, "Xylitol Administered Only During Respiratory Infections Failed to Prevent Acute Otitis Media." *Pediatrics* 109(2002): 19.

Tufts University School of Dental Medicine: Dry Mouth, 1986, 13. Makinen, KK, Soderling E. "Solubility of Calcium salts, enamel, and hydroxyapatite in queous soultions of simple carbohydrates." *Calcif. Tissue Int.* (1984)36: 64–71.

Uhari, M, T Kontiokari, and M Niemelä. "A Novel Use of Xylitol Sugar in Preventing Acute Otitis Media." *Pediatrics* 102(1998): 879–884.

Uhari, M, T Kontiokari, M Koskela, and Marjo Niemelä. "Xylitol chewing gum in prevention of acute otitis media: double blind randomised trial." *BMJ* 313(1996): 1180–1183.

WHO/FAO Evaluation of certain food additives and contaminants, Twenty-seventh Report of the joint FAO/WHO Expert Committee on Food Additives, Geneva, WHO Technical Report Series No. 696, 1983.

Wright, Peter. "Xylitol Sugar and Acute Otitis Media." *Pediatrics* 102(1998): 971–972.

Index

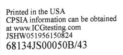

9 781681 628196